BY A. DUGAN AND THE EDITORS OF CONSUMER GUIDE®

FOR MEN ONLY

FLATTEN your STOMACH

Louis Weber, President
Publications International, Ltd.
3841 West Oakton Street
Skokie, Illinois 60076

Permission is never granted for commercial purposes.

Manufactured in the United States of America
10 9 8 7 6

Library of Congress Catalog Card Number: 83-63051

ISBN: 0-88176-179-6

Cover design: Linda Snow Shum
Book design: Karen A. Yops
Photography: Sam Griffith Studios
Model: Bill Carel

Contents

THE 7-DAY PROGRAM —————— 4

This 7-Day Flatten Your Stomach Program has a different exercise routine for every day of the week. Follow it faithfully and you'll see results fast.

DAY 1 ————————————— 8

Get into your exercise gear and let's get to work. You're on your way to a physique that's sleek, trim, and hard.

DAY 2 ————————————— 16

Don't stop if Day 1 made you a little sore. Day 2 will warm up those muscles and help work out the kinks.

DAY 3 ————————————— 24

As you go through Day 3, notice which muscles are doing the work and try to concentrate your efforts there.

DAY 4 ————————————— 32

You've made it to the midpoint of the program. Don't slack off now. You're already stronger.

DAY 5 ————————————— 40

Remember that the warm up and cool down are essential to the program. Don't neglect them.

DAY 6 ————————————— 48

Every day you're working a little harder, and every day you're closer to your goal.

DAY 7 ————————————— 56

Arrive at Day 7, and you should already be aware of changes: tighter muscles, more energy, a trimmer torso.

THE 7-DAY PROGRAM

Not too many years ago the picture of success included a paunch. A prosperous gentleman looked, well, portly and substantial. His waistcoats were double-breasted and often sported a gold watch chain draped across an expanse of abdomen that bespoke satisfaction and abundance. But no more. Today it's a trim, flat stomach that sends out to the world a message of youth, health, vitality, and success. Excessive girth has come to be recognized as a health hazard, and it can be a social and professional hindrance as well.

While there's no doubt that a flat stomach is desirable, it's not necessarily easy to achieve. Unless we make a special effort, most of us simply don't get the kind of exercise needed to maintain a fit, trim body. Even if you keep your weight down and participate in some form of sports or aerobic activity regularly, your stomach may bulge and sag because the abdominal muscles themselves haven't been toned.

The four layers of muscle that sheathe the abdomen are relatively thin, yet they have several important functions. They protect, support, and contain the hollow organs of the abdominal cavity, and they help to keep the pelvis in proper alignment, thereby helping us maintain upright posture. When these muscles are untoned, the abdomen sags forward, and the back of the pelvis may begin to tilt upward. This causes the lower vertebrae to rotate forward, resulting in a "swayback." Because the vertebrae are out of alignment, they press against one another, leading to lower back pain. It's a triple curse—bulging belly, bad posture, and back pain.

Luckily these muscles usually respond rapidly to exercise. But a marathon of sit-ups and toe touches—two exercises often thought to flatten the stomach—is likely to overdevelop certain abdominal muscles at the expense of others. Your abdomen may be hard, but it probably won't be flat. A trim abdomen and midriff requires a balanced program of exercises designed to tone the muscle layers that mold the abdomen.

The Abdominal Muscles

Each of the four abdominal muscles functions in a different movement. The outermost layer, the *rectus abdominis,* is primarily a flexor; its fibers run vertically from the rib cage to the pelvic bone. To feel this muscle, lie on the floor, knees bent, feet flat, head raised. Now touch your upper abdomen. That hard layer is the *rectus abdominis.*

The next layer is the *external oblique,* a broad thin muscle that originates at the borders of the lower eight ribs and runs obliquely forward and downward. To feel it, place your hands at your waist and bend to the side; you should be able to feel the external oblique tighten up. Running underneath the external oblique is the *internal oblique.* Its fibers start at the hip and run obliquely upward to meet the lower ribs. This muscle is too deep to be easily seen or felt, but its action is apparent when you "suck in" to button a too-tight pair of pants.

The fibers of the innermost muscle, the *transverse abdominis,* run across the abdomen from side to side. Although it is also too deep to be easily seen or felt, when it is untoned its effects are all too evident as a pot belly.

In order to be effective an exercise program must evenly tone all these muscles, and that's exactly the way this Flatten Your Stomach program has been designed. Our routines carefully alternate the muscles exercised so that each reaches a peak of toning. If you follow the program carefully, you'll have a flatter stomach and a trimmer waistline.

The Seven-Day Program

This is a seven-day program, with a different routine for every day. You may choose to work out every day or every other day. Of course, the less frequently you exercise, the more slowly you'll shape up. Don't exercise less frequently than every other day. After only 72 hours without exercise, your fitness level begins to decline. That means that any gains you've made begin to disappear. If you do let more than two days pass without exercising, drop back to an earlier routine and build up to your former level.

These routines are progressively more difficult. If you prefer you could repeat the same routine until you feel you've mastered it and then progress to the following routine. Don't stay at the same level for more than two to three weeks, though. For peak training effects to occur, a muscle must be made to work continually harder.

If at any time, an exercise begins to seem easy to you, add from three to five repetitions the next time you do that exercise. As written, each routine should take 30 minutes or less. As you add repetitions, it will take a little longer.

Warm Ups and Cool Downs

Each routine contains a warm up and a cool down. Each is essential to the success of your program. Don't neglect the warm up and cool down.

A warm up gets your body going. It loosens up the muscles all over your body and gets your heart and lungs working faster. Warm ups make your muscle-toning exercise more effective. As your body temperature rises slightly, the blood supply to your muscles increases and the rate and force of muscle contractions also increase. You'll get more out of the effort you put into your workout.

Warm ups also make you less prone to injury during exercise. They stretch the ligaments and connective tissues to permit greater flexibility and lessen the chance of muscle tears and sprains.

After you've completed the muscle-toning exercises in your routine, you need to give your body a chance to cool down. Cool downs help your muscles begin to relax. They allow your circulatory system to slow down gradually. A proper cool down will help minimize soreness and stiffness and will help you wind down after your routine, leaving you feeling relaxed and pleasantly loose.

If you have a minute or two to spare, try these simple stretches for the lower back after our cool downs. They're a double dose of relaxation. Stand with your feet comfortably apart, arms hanging loosely at your sides. Slowly roll your head and torso forward and hang limply for a count of 20. Slowly straighten up. Raise one knee, clasp it with both hands and pull it to your chest. Lower your head toward your knee and hold for a count of five, then lower your knee. Repeat with other knee.

The Exercises Themselves

Our exercises for the stomach are a combination of spot exercises and stretches. These spot exercises are muscle-toners, not so-called "spot-reducers." Exercising one part of the body will not reduce the amount of fat in that area. However, exercise can change the shape of a body area by restoring muscle tone. An untoned muscle is flabby and soft. Restoring the muscle's tone through exercise will give it a firm and attractive shape.

Some exercises end with stretches, particularly when the exercise has put a lot of stress on a certain muscle group. When a muscle works, it contracts. Its fibers shorten and bulk up. Stretches counteract the effects of stress on muscles by helping them and their connective tissues to relax and lengthen. If the body's connective tissues aren't stretched frequently, they can become tight and may limit your range of movement. If not stretched at all for a long time, the tissues may snap, causing injury and pain. Do the stretches slowly, and don't stretch any farther than is comfortable. Eventually, you will be looser and more flexible and will be able to stretch farther.

The stomach-flattening exercises are carefully designed to help your muscles develop evenly. This even development of all the abdominal muscles is what gives you the shape you're after. Our exercise routines carefully alternate the muscles used. Do them in the sequence given for the greatest benefit.

Making It Work

Following these guidelines will help make your exercise program more enjoyable, keep you free from injury, and ensure your success.

• Dress comfortably—shorts and a T-shirt or a light exercise suit—in clothing that allows heat loss. Don't wear any plastic or rubberized suits.

• Wear running shoes during the warm ups to protect the feet, knees, and ankles. Kick off your shoes for the exercises if that's more comfortable for you.

• If possible, work on a wooden floor or on carpet. You want a surface that gives with the body. For floor exercises, work on a mat, or put a carpet remnant, a piece of foam rubber, or a folded towel under your lower back to prevent irritation.

• Try to exercise at least four times a week, more often if possible.

• Establish an exercise schedule. You shouldn't exercise just before bedtime or just after eating. Most any other time is fine. Once you choose the best time, stick to it. Making exercise a habit makes it easier for you and offers the greatest rewards.

• Follow the routines carefully. They've been designed to tone and shape muscles properly and avoid injury.

• If you cannot do an exercise exactly as described, don't worry. Try it, and then continue with the routine. As your strength and flexibility increase, your performance will improve.

• Don't push yourself past your body's limits. Body structure and flexibility vary greatly from person to person. The structure of your joints or the length of your limbs may prevent you from stretching as far as our model.

• As you work through each day's routine, keep moving. Avoid taking long breaks between exercises, but don't rush through the routine either. Work at a steady pace; your body should feel like it's working hard, but not that it's in an endurance contest. Putting on some lively music while you exercise may help.

• If you're winded or breathless, or if you suffer side stitches, pain, or weakness, take a little break. Count to five and catch your breath. If you feel tightness or pain in the chest, stop exercising and consult your physician.

• You may feel a little sore or stiff the first few days that you exercise, especially if you haven't exercised for a while. Don't stop exercising, but take it easy. As you become stronger and more flexible, the soreness and stiffness will disappear. Remember too that proper warm ups and cool downs help minimize soreness.

• Be careful of your back. The abdominal muscles work with the muscles of the back to support the torso. Therefore, some exercises for the abdomen may also put strain on the back. These exercises will strengthen the back gradually, but go slowly at first, especially if your back is weak. If you experience back pain during an exercise, stop for a few seconds, count to five, then pull one knee (or both if you're doing floor exercises) to the chest. Hold for a few seconds, then continue your routine.

• Don't be discouraged if you gain a little weight in the beginning of this program. A small weight gain means more muscle, not more fat. Your muscles are becoming firmer, denser, harder, and heavier. Those few extra pounds will disappear after another week or two of regular exercise.

• This program was developed in consultation with medical experts. However, it is recommended that you consult your doctor before beginning this or any exercise program.

A Note About Fat and Flab

When a body's out of shape, there are usually two kinds of problems. One is fat, and the other is flab. Flab is untoned muscle tissue, and it's the target of this Flatten Your Stomach program. These exercises are designed to tone and firm muscles that haven't been worked for a while.

To achieve top form, most people also need to lose a little excess fat. Fat isn't all bad. It insulates the body against physical trauma; it protects, cushions, and supports your internal organs; and it is a highly efficient source of fuel. Excess fat, however, is another story. An excessive amount of body fat makes you look bad, and it impairs your health.

Most people now realize that in order to lose weight you have to expend more calories than you consume, but most people deal with only one side of that equation. They consume fewer calories. Unfortunately, when you cut your calorie intake your body satisfies its energy needs by taking from muscle tissue as well as fat. Muscle burns more calories than fat. Therefore, once you've lost some weight, your body will need fewer calories throughout your daily activities—you'll be more prone to putting on weight than you were before you dieted. If you go on a crash diet, the situation gets even worse. When suddenly deprived of calories, the body decides that it had better hold the line and conserve as much energy as possible. It slows down your metabolic rate to burn fewer calories than before. Even as you struggle

to take weight off, the body fights mightily to hold on to what it already has.

But let's take a look at what happens when you combine dieting with exercise to achieve weight loss. For some as yet undetermined reason, when you reduce your calorie intake and increase your activity level, the body decides to concentrate on your fat stores to supply its energy needs. The pounds you drop will be mostly fat, leaving you with a higher percentage of calorie-consuming muscle. Furthermore, vigorous exercise that gets your heart and lungs pumping harder for at least 30 minutes increases your metabolic rate for some time after you've completed exercising. You'll burn more calories sitting around watching television after your workout than you would have if you hadn't exercised at all.

It seems obvious that the way to go to lose weight is both to restrict your calorie intake and increase your activity level. Followed faithfully, this Flatten Your Stomach program is a step in the right direction. However, if you have more than a little to lose, you'll probably want to speed up the process. So try to be more active generally. Use the stairs instead of the elevator; ride your bike to work, relax with a brisk walk instead of a beer after supper. For the fastest results of all, supplement the Flatten Your Stomach program with a half hour of aerobic activity at least three times a week. Aerobic activities like running, swimming, cycling, and rowing are the greatest calorie-burners of exercise and they'll benefit your body in lots of other ways, too.

Let's Get Started

That's all you need to know to get going on the Flatten Your Stomach program. Why not start right now? Get into some comfortable clothes, put on some upbeat music, and turn the page. You'll look better by next week.

TRACK TAKE-OFF

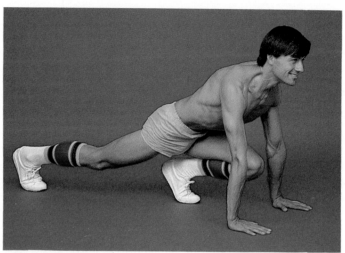

Starting Position

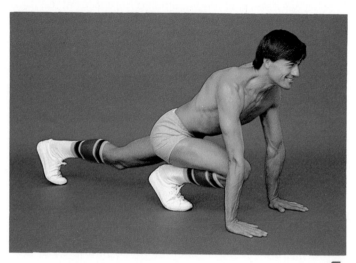

A

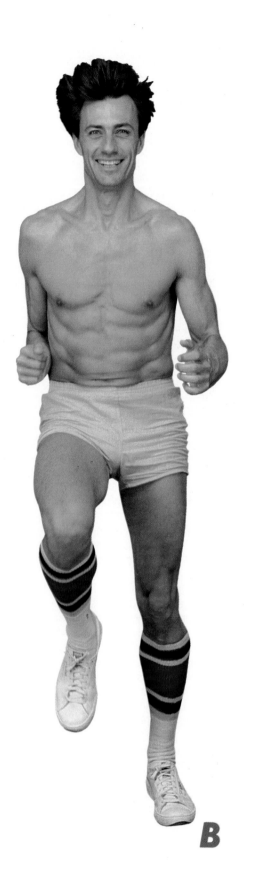

A Without moving hands from floor, "run" by rapidly reversing leg positions for 20 counts.

B Arise and run in place for 50 counts, lifting knees high. Keep your mouth open and breathe!

B

TWO-POINT SHOT

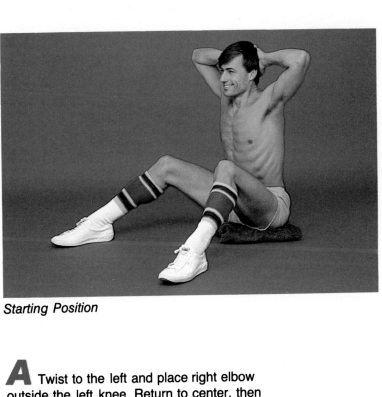

Starting Position

A Twist to the left and place right elbow outside the left knee. Return to center, then twist to the right and place left elbow outside the right knee. Repeat 5 times to each side.

A

TWO MORE POINTS

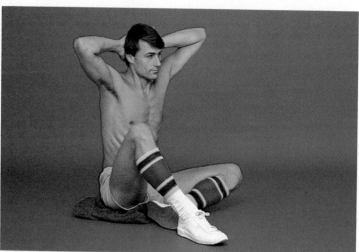

Starting Position

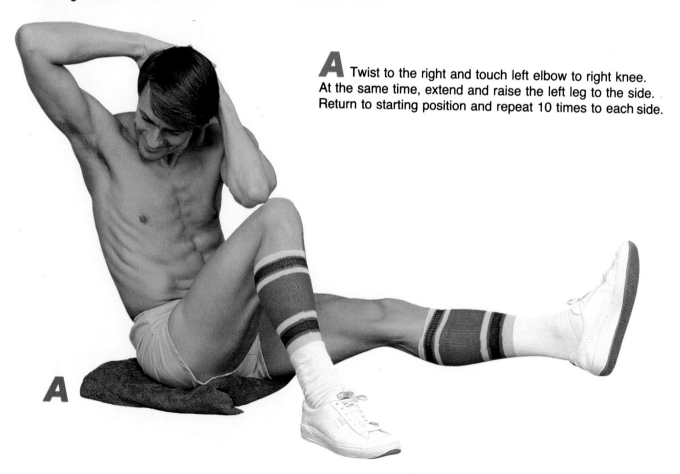

A Twist to the right and touch left elbow to right knee. At the same time, extend and raise the left leg to the side. Return to starting position and repeat 10 times to each side.

A

STRIKE OUT

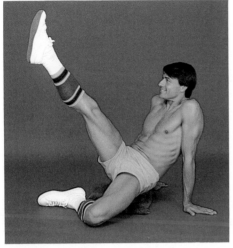

Starting Position

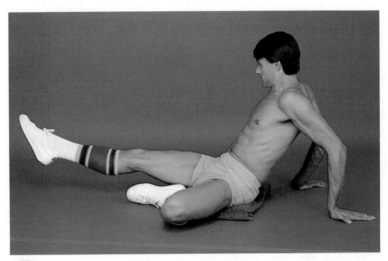

A

A Circle the right leg toward the floor, simultaneously lowering hips to the floor.

B Raise hips as you arc the leg upward. Make 10 circles with each leg.

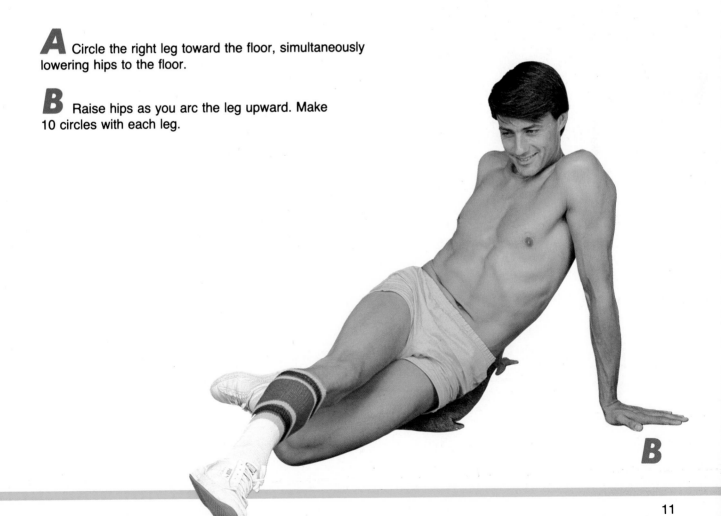

B

SWING THROUGH

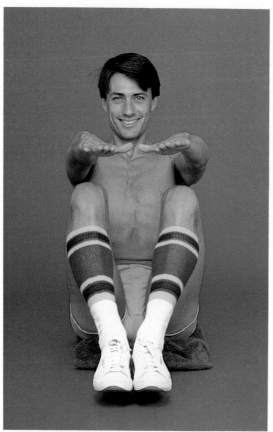

Starting Position

A Extend legs to the left, swinging arms to the right at the same time. Bring the knees back in to the chest, then extend legs to the right, swinging arms to the left. Keep feet off the floor throughout the movement. Repeat 10 times to each side.

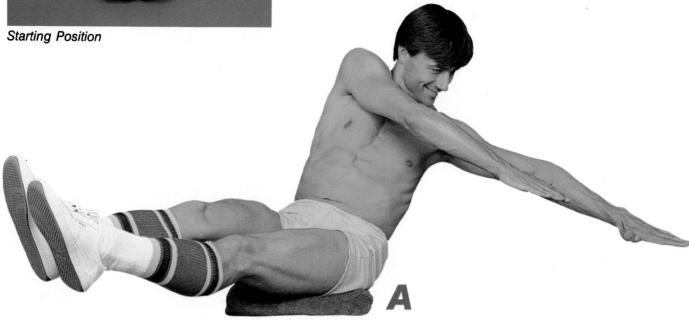

A

12

SQUEEZE PLAY

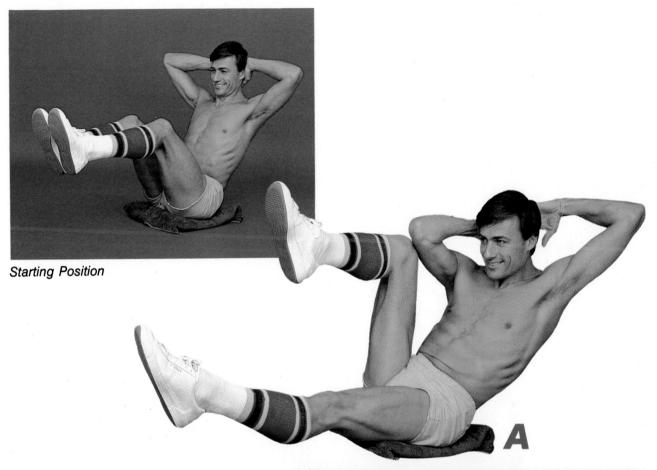

Starting Position

A Pull the right knee in toward the chest, bringing right elbow forward to touch the knee. At the same time extend left leg, keeping it off the floor. Try to keep the lower part of each leg parallel to the floor throughout the movement. Repeat 10 times, alternating right-left.

B Continue the leg movement, but touch elbow to opposite knee—right elbow to left knee, left elbow to right knee. Repeat 10 times, alternating left-right.

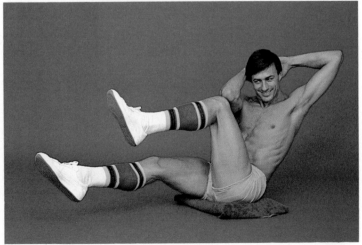

OVERKILL

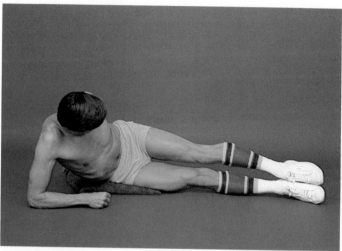

Starting Position

A Lift both legs off the floor as high as possible. Raise right arm and try to touch feet. Repeat 10 times on each side.

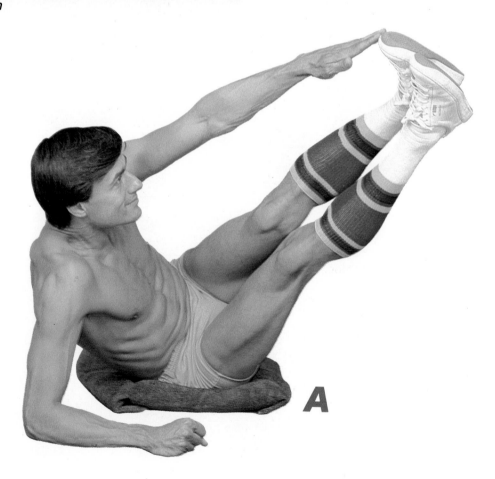

A

FLY OUT

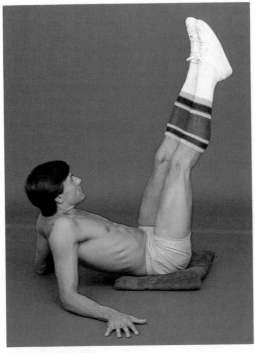

Starting Position

A Lower both legs to the floor on the right. Raise legs back to center position, then lower them to the left. Repeat 10 times.

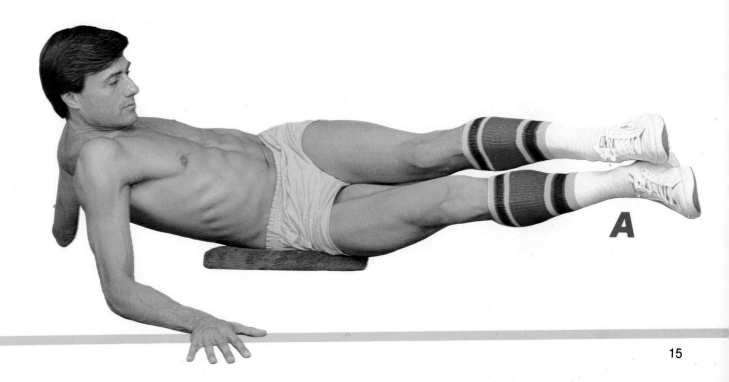

DAY 2 — Warm Up

POWER PLAY

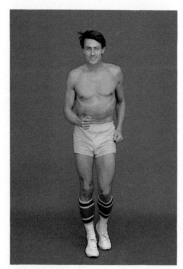

Starting Position

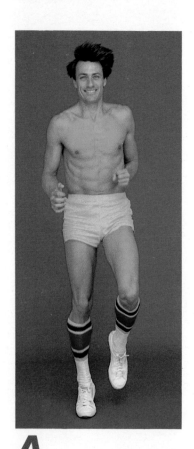

A

A Run in place for 75 counts, lifting knees high.

B Don't stop—put hands on hips and hop on one foot for 15 counts, then on the other for 15 counts.

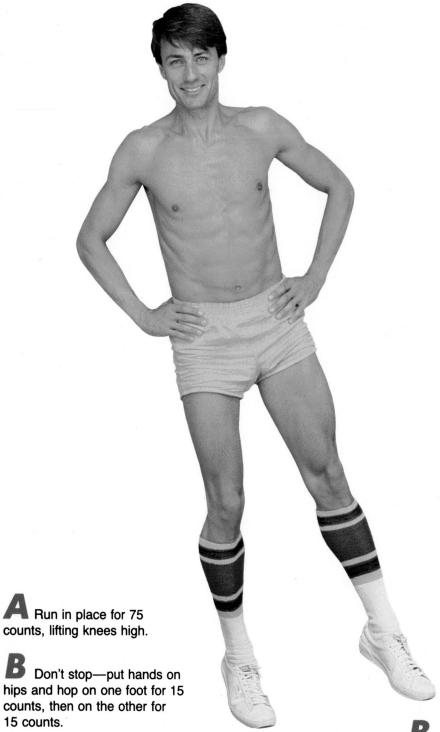

B

LOVE HANDLE ELIMINATOR

A Kick right leg up and to the side, simultaneously swinging arms from the left toward the right leg. Lower the leg, return arms to starting position, and repeat 10 times on each side.

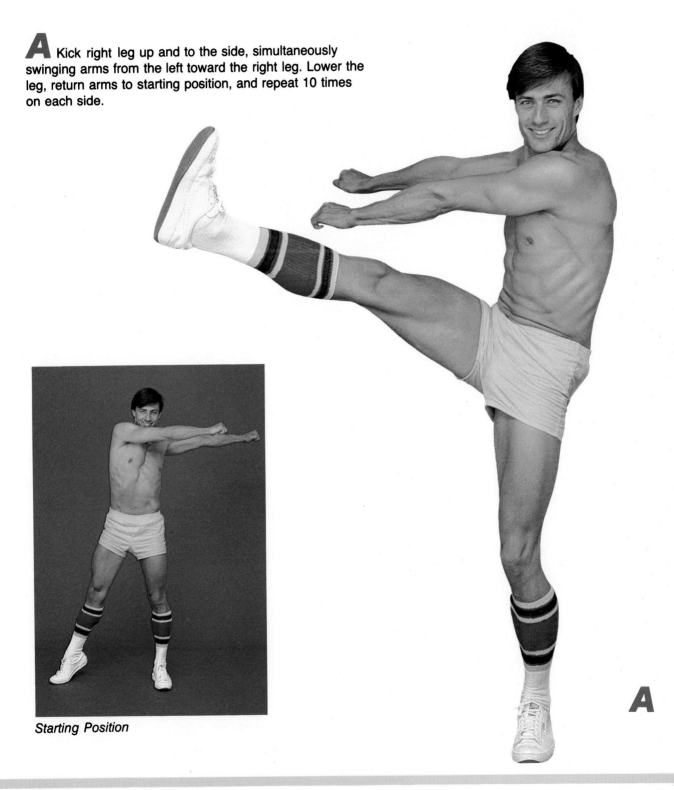

Starting Position

A

OFF SIDES

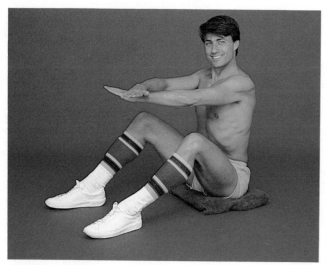

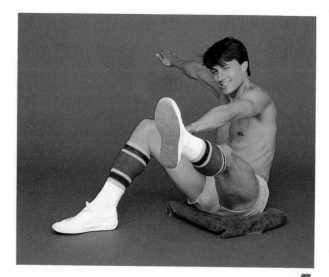

Starting Position

A

A Extend left leg up and to the left. At the same time, swing arms out to the sides and touch left leg with left hand. Return to starting position. Repeat 10 times to the left and 10 times to the right.

B Don't stop. Repeat the exercise, but this time alternate sides—first extend the left leg, then the right—for a count of 20.

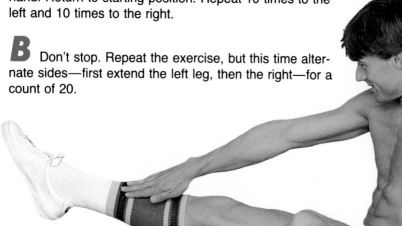

B

POP UP

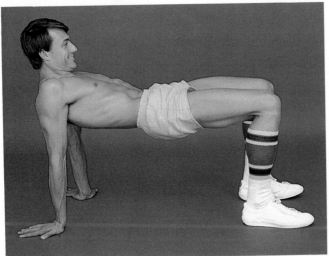

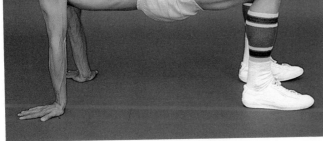

Starting Position

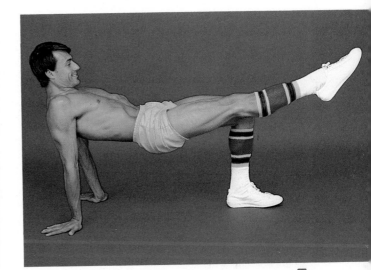

A

A Extend right leg forward from the hip.

B Swing right leg out to the side as far as possible, then back to the forward position. Repeat 10 times with each leg.

B

LIFT OFF

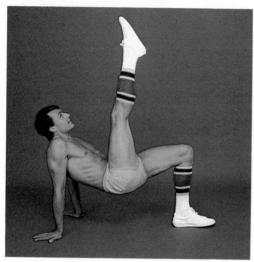

Starting Position

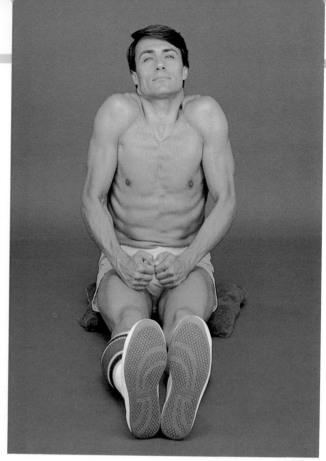

B

A Describe a circle with the right leg: Swing it down toward the floor, then arc it back up to the starting position. Make 10 circles with each leg.

B To release tension in the arms and shoulders, sit with legs extended forward. Make fists and squeeze tightly, simultaneously lifting shoulders toward the ears. Hold 5 counts. Relax. Repeat 3 times.

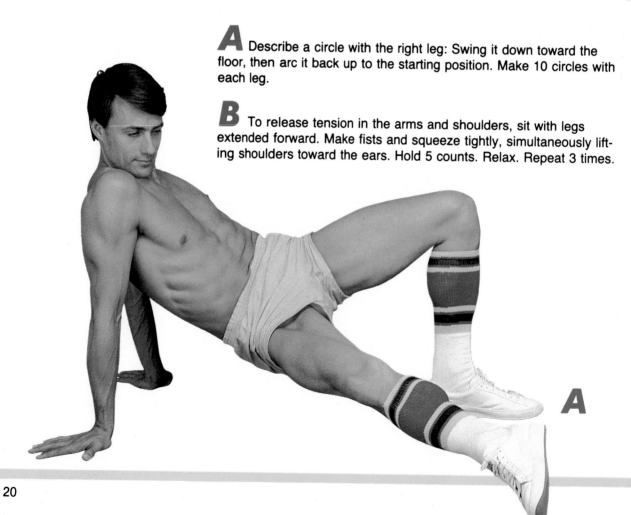

A

SQUEEZE PLAY PLUS

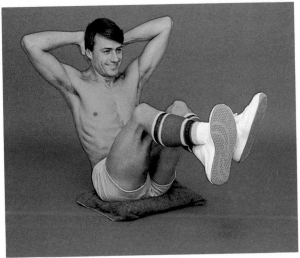

Starting Position

A Bring knees in toward chest and press elbows forward to touch knees. Return knees and elbows to starting position. (The movement is tuck-release, tuck-release). Repeat 10 times.

B Sit with soles together, hands on ankles. Pull head and chest toward the ankles. Hold for 5 counts. This will stretch the connective tissues of the back. It should feel great! Repeat 3 times.

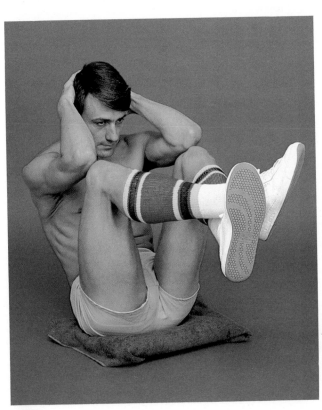

A

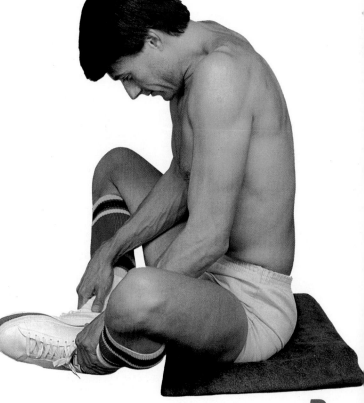

B

STRIKE OUT #1

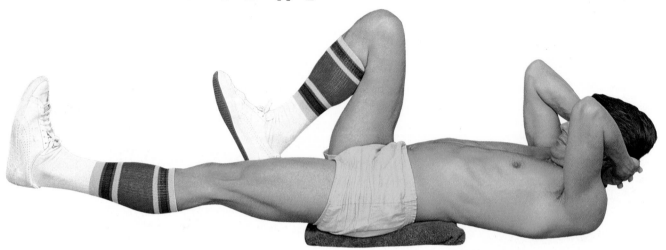

Starting Position

A Slowly extend the bent leg forward, keeping the foot flexed. Do not lower either foot to floor. Bend leg back in to chest. Repeat 5 times with each leg. Lower both legs to floor and rest for a count of 5. Then repeat exercise, once again extending each leg 5 times.

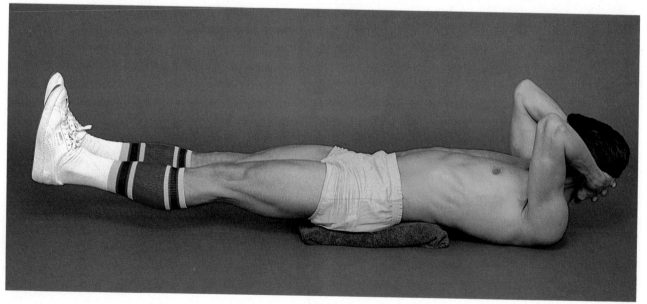

A

STRIKE OUT #2

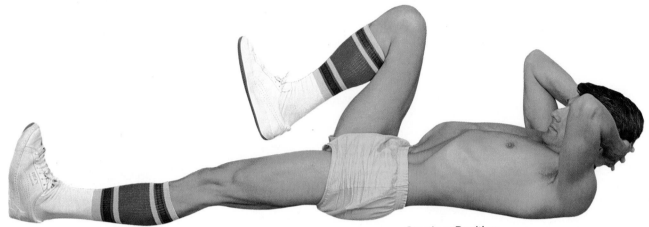

Starting Position

A Keeping the foot flexed and without touching the floor, extend the bent leg forward. Bring it back to starting position. Repeat 10 times with each leg.

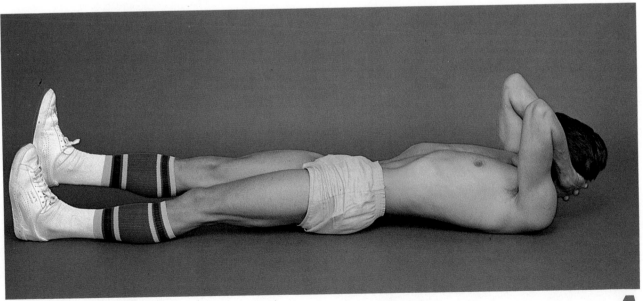

A

JUMPIN' JACK

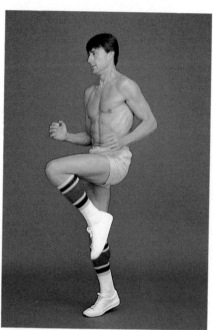

Starting Position

A Run in place for 100 counts.

B Jump in place for 50 counts, pumping arms back and forth for increased vigor.

B

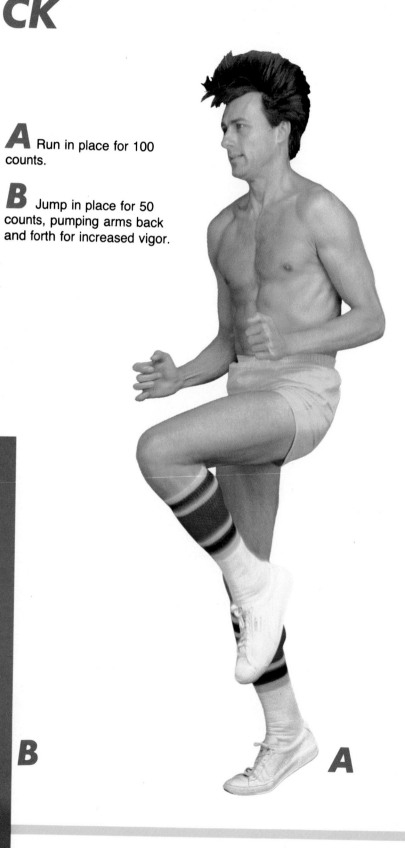

A

Warm Up

TORSO TWIST

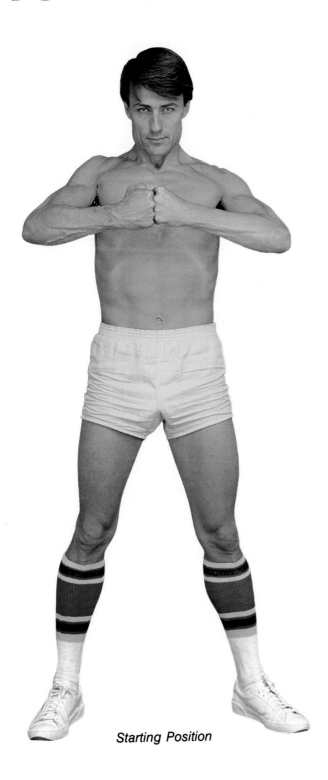

Starting Position

A While pressing knuckles together, twist upper torso quickly from side to side. Twist to each side 10 times.

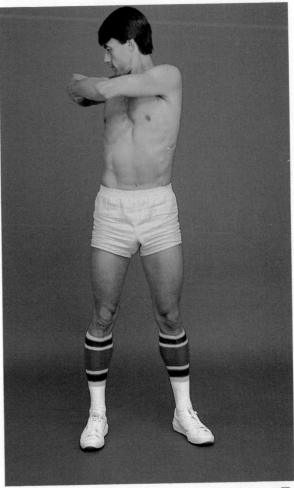

A

25

SWING IT LOW

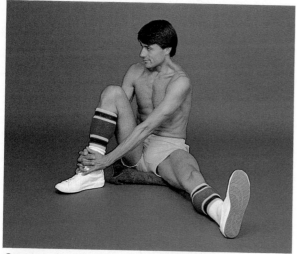

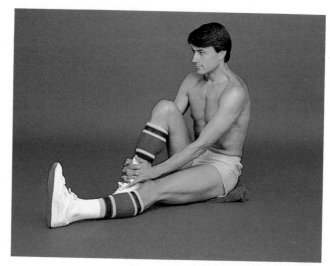

Starting Position

A

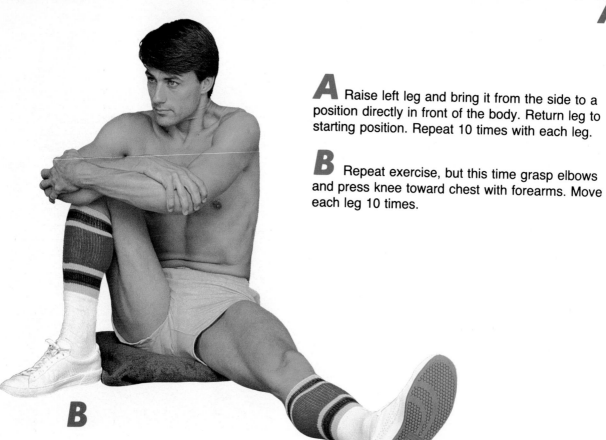

B

A Raise left leg and bring it from the side to a position directly in front of the body. Return leg to starting position. Repeat 10 times with each leg.

B Repeat exercise, but this time grasp elbows and press knee toward chest with forearms. Move each leg 10 times.

THE BIG HEIST

A Lift hip and raise extended leg straight up.

B Lower leg toward floor and out to the side, then swing it forward to return to starting position. Repeat 10 times with each leg.

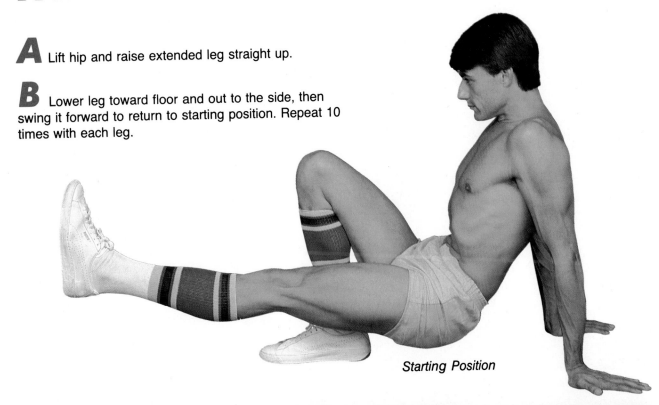

Starting Position

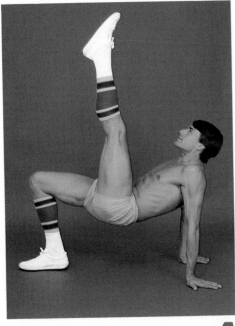

A

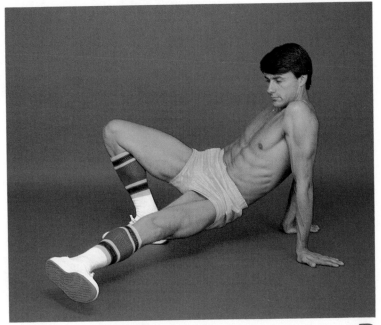

B

THE KICKER

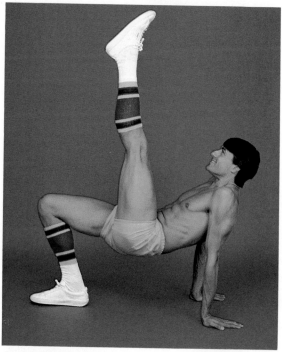

Starting Position

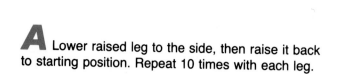

A

B

A Lower raised leg to the side, then raise it back to starting position. Repeat 10 times with each leg.

B Sit with legs extended forward, arms hanging at sides, hands turned back and resting on the floor. Shrug shoulders forward and allow head to hang loosely. Hold 5 counts. Repeat 3 times.

SUPER TIGHT

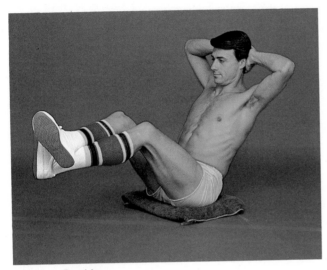

Starting Position

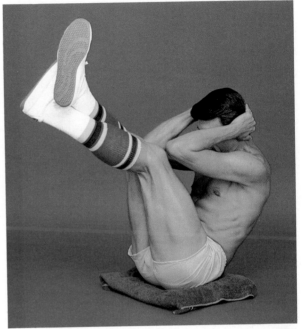

A

A Raise and straighten legs as much as possible, pressing elbows forward to touch knees. Release, return to starting position, and repeat 10 times.

B Lie on your back with legs extended forward. Bend one knee up, clasp it with both hands, and pull toward chest as hard as possible. Lift head and pull toward knee. Hold 5 counts. Release and repeat with other knee. This will release tension in the lower back.

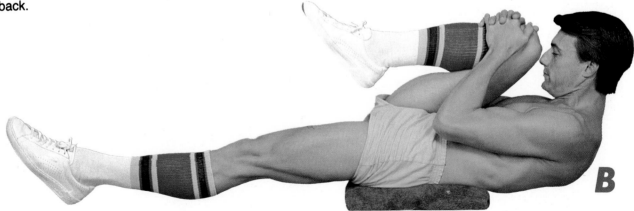

B

CATCH IT

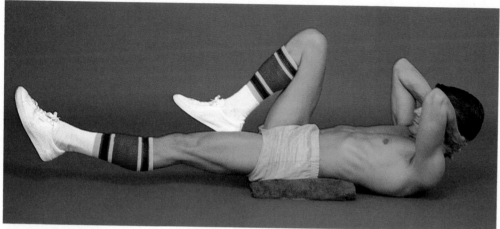

Starting Position

A Keeping the left leg off the floor, extend the right leg straight up, then slowly lower it to meet the left leg. Hold 3 counts. Then bend right knee in toward body. Repeat 10 times with each leg.

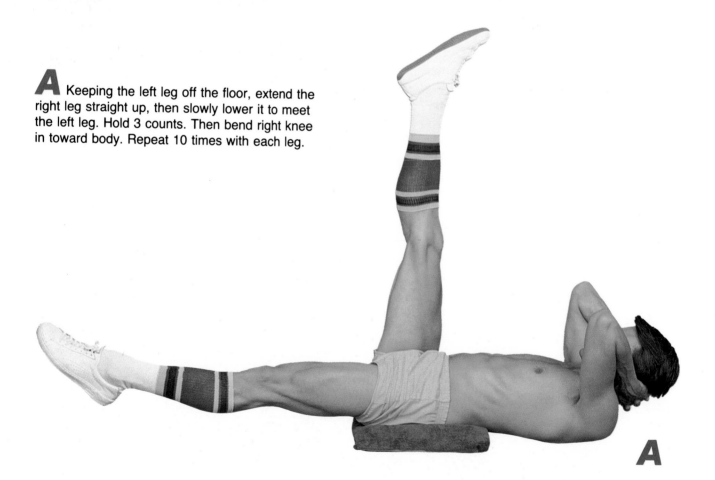

A

TEXAS LEAGUER

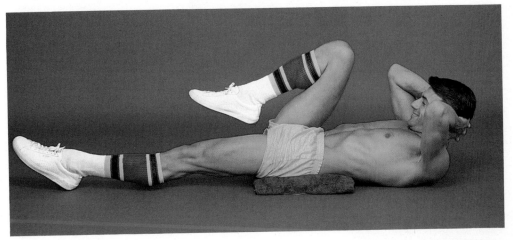

Starting Position

A Extend the right leg straight up.

B Slowly lower right leg to line up with left leg on the floor. Bend right knee in toward body. Repeat 10 times with each leg.

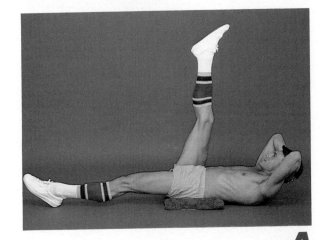

A

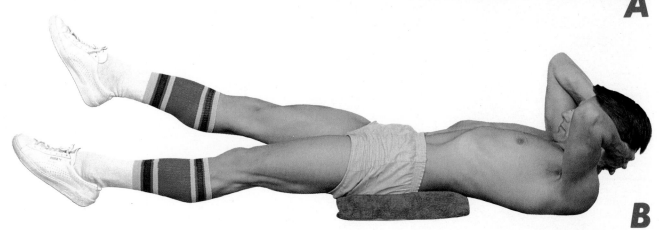

B

TOUCHDOWN

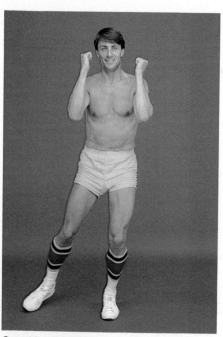

Starting Position

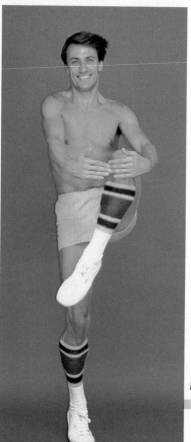

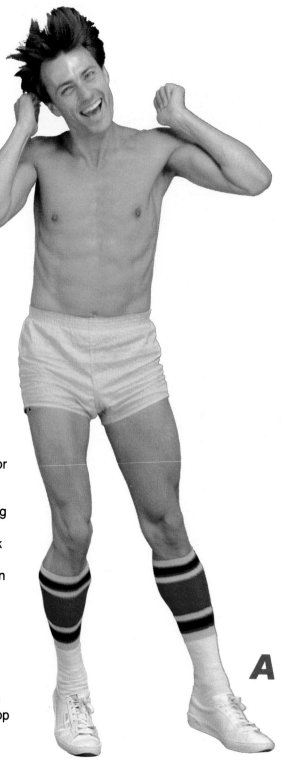

A Kick side to side for 50 counts: Kick left leg out to side and back to center, then kick right leg out to side and back to center. Pump arms back and forth for added aerobic benefit. Then run in place for 125 counts.

B Hop 10 times on right leg, lifting left knee toward chest with each hop. Encircle the lifted knee with arms, opening arms to sides as you drop the knee. Repeat on left leg.

B

A

TOTAL CONTROL

A Bend left leg and bring right elbow down to touch left knee, at the same time swinging left arm up and back. Repeat 10 times on each side.

B Stand with arms at sides. Twist torso from side to side swinging arms up and back loosely as you twist. You should feel a pull in the torso, but no strain. Twist to each side 10 times.

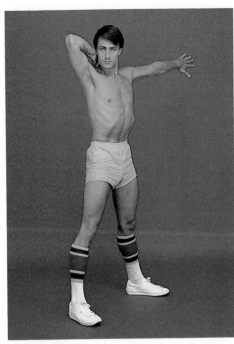

Starting Position

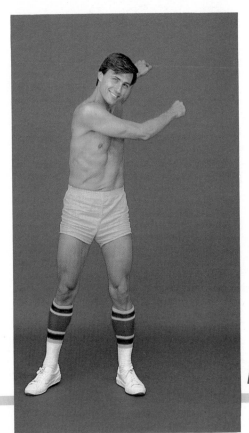

B

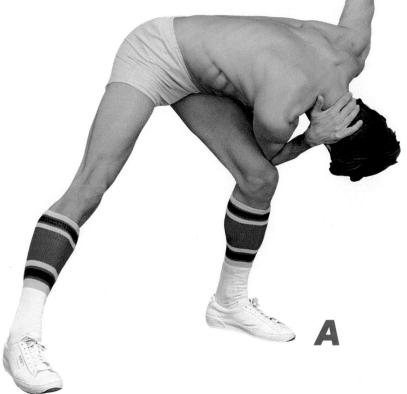

A

OFF SIDE

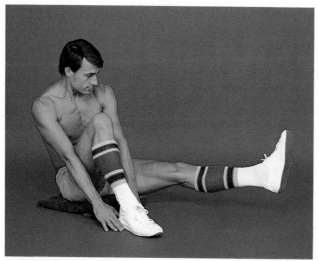

Starting Position

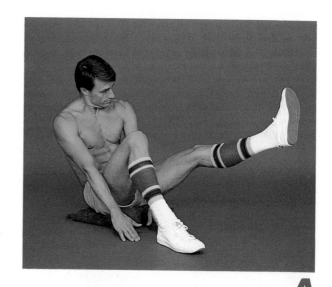

A

A Lift the extended leg as high as possible, then lower almost but not quite to the floor. Repeat 5 times. Then move hands a few inches closer to torso, and again lift and lower the extended leg 5 times.

B Move hands closer to torso. Lift and lower extended leg 5 times. Repeat entire sequence with other leg.

B

SUPER OFF SIDE

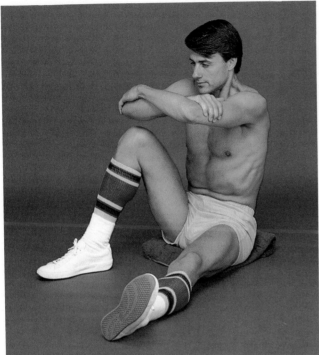

Starting Position

A Raise the extended leg off the floor as high as possible, bringing forearms down to touch the raised knee. Lower leg to floor. Repeat 10 times on each side.

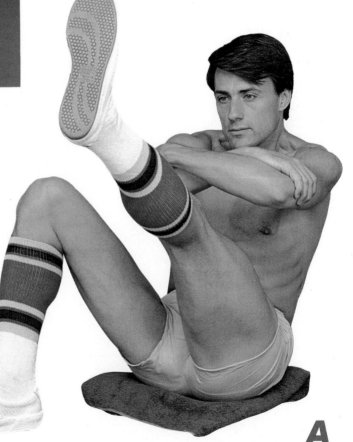

A

ROUGHING THE KICKER

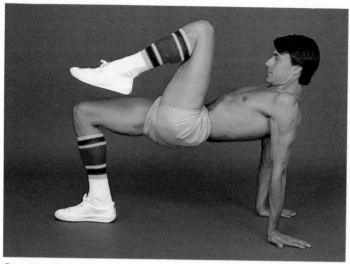

Starting Position

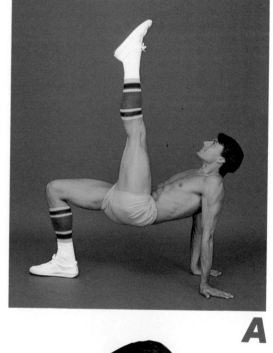

A

A Extend the left leg straight up, then lower it back to starting position near the chest.

B Extend the left leg directly out to the side, then bring it back close to the chest as in the starting position. Repeat 10 times on each side.

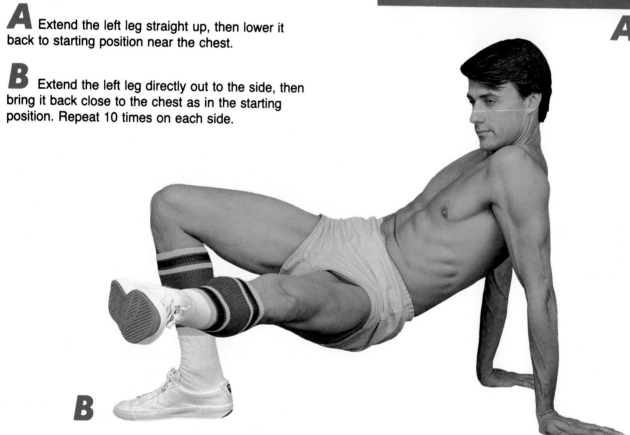

B

MORE ROUGHING THE KICKER

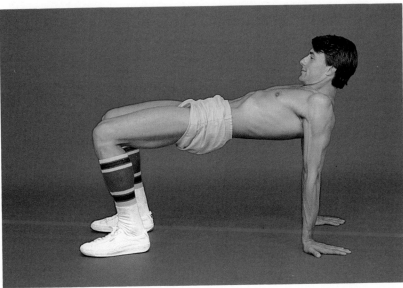

Starting Position

A Raise the left leg straight up and bring right hand to touch left ankle. Return to starting position. Repeat 10 times on each side.

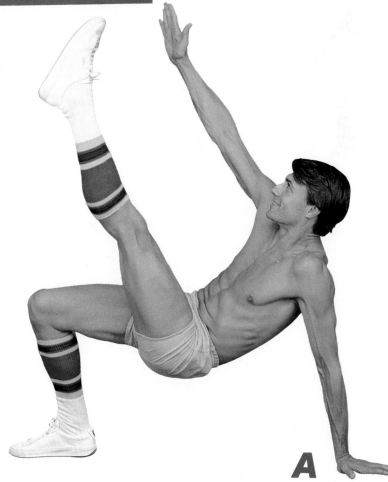

A

GETTING STRONG NOW

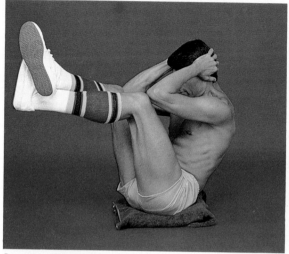

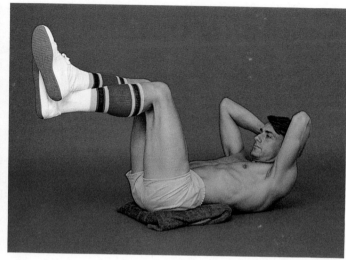

Starting Position

A

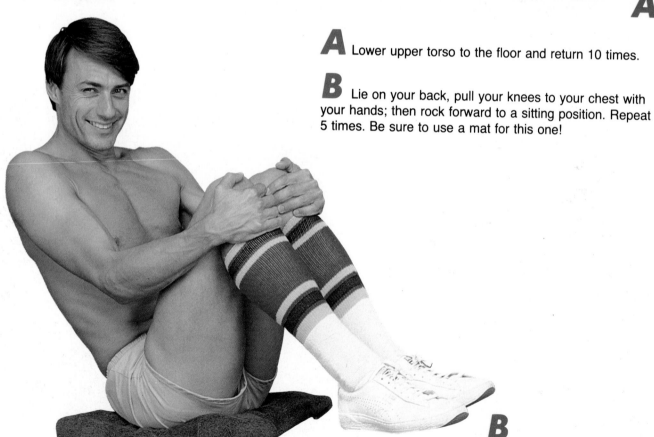

A Lower upper torso to the floor and return 10 times.

B Lie on your back, pull your knees to your chest with your hands; then rock forward to a sitting position. Repeat 5 times. Be sure to use a mat for this one!

B

SIDE UP

A Raise the right leg as high as possible and touch it with left elbow. Lower leg. Repeat 5 times on each side.

B Return to starting position. Raise right leg as high as possible toward the center. Lower. Repeat 10 times on each side.

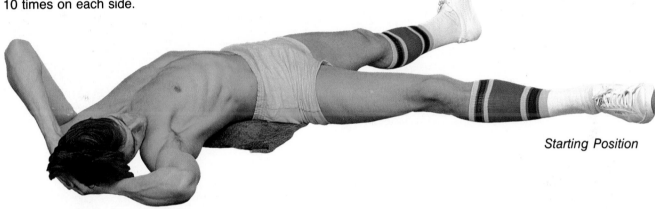

Starting Position

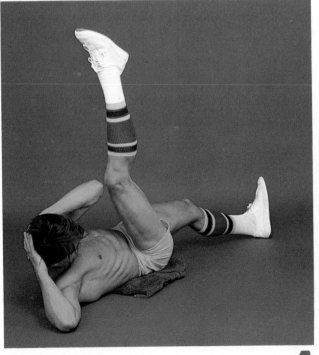

A

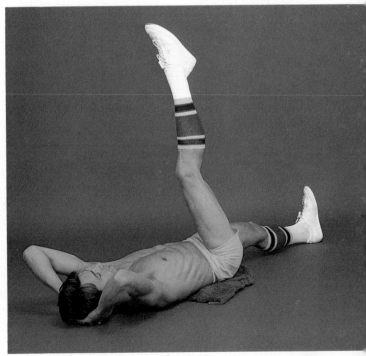

B

DAY 5 — Warm Up

LEAD OFF

A Run in place for 150 counts, kicking up your heels in back and swinging the opposite arm forward with each step.

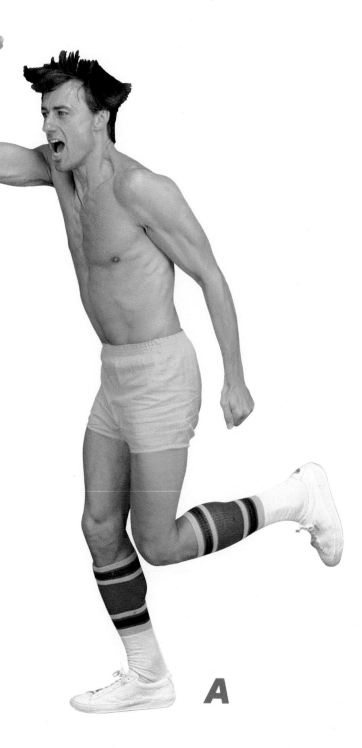

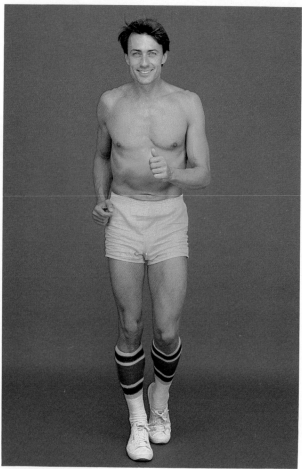

Starting Position

HIGH DIVE

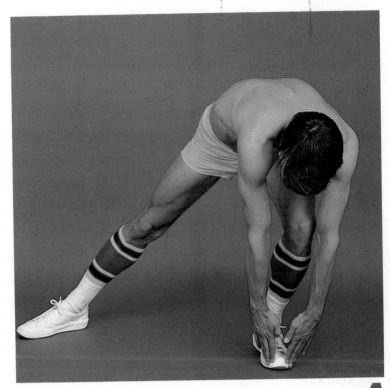

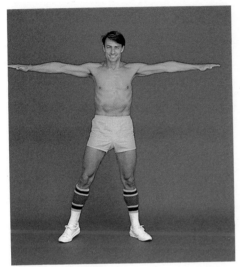

Starting Position

A

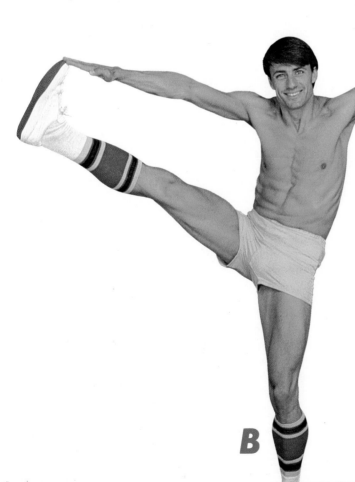

B

A Bend left knee, keeping right leg straight; lower torso and touch both hands to left toe.

B Straighten left knee, raise torso, swing arms out to the sides, and lift right leg to the side as high as possible. Touch right hand to right foot. Lower right leg to return to starting position. The entire action should be one continuous, springy movement. Repeat 10 times on each side.

SPARE

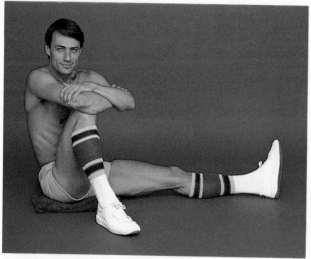

Starting Position

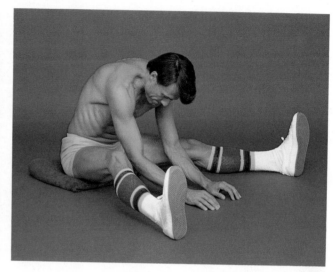

B

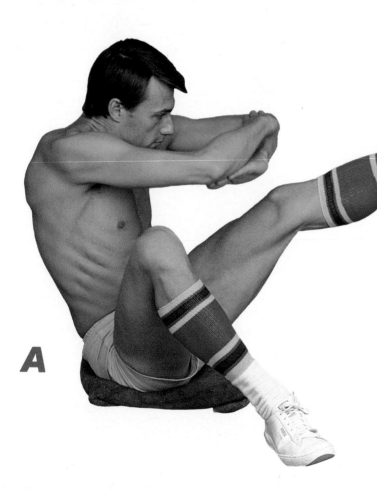

A

A Raise the left leg and try to touch forearms to left shin. Lower leg. Repeat 10 times on each side.

B Sit on floor with legs wide apart. Place hands as far forward on floor as possible, then slowly bend elbows toward floor. Hold for 10 counts. This stretch will help maintain flexibility in the back.

BLITZ SIDE

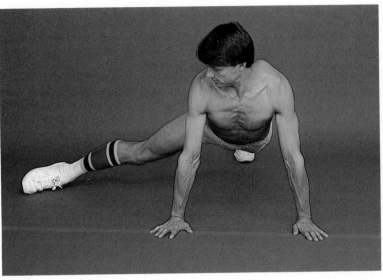

Starting Position

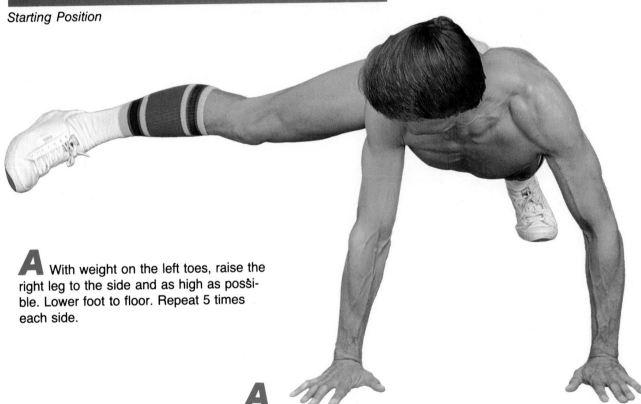

A With weight on the left toes, raise the right leg to the side and as high as possible. Lower foot to floor. Repeat 5 times each side.

A

BLITZ SIDE PLUS

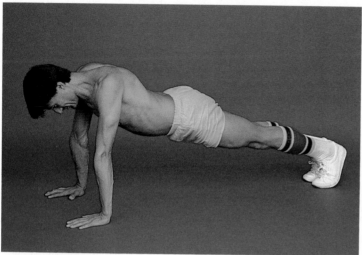

Starting Position

A Swing the left leg forward and touch left foot with left hand. Swing left leg back, but do not let it touch the floor. Swing left arm forward and up. Repeat 10 times on each side.

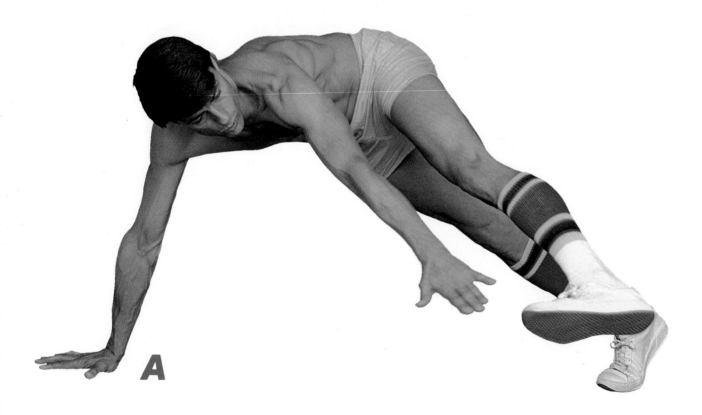

A

GETTING EVEN STRONGER

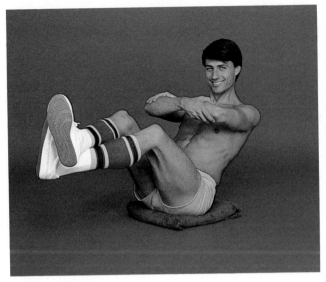

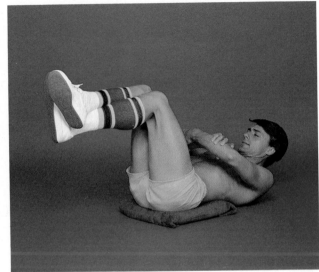

Starting Position

A Lower the upper torso to the floor and return 10 times.

B Sit with legs wide apart. Press right fist into right armpit and raise left arm overhead. Bend torso to the right. Hold 5 counts. Repeat on opposite side.

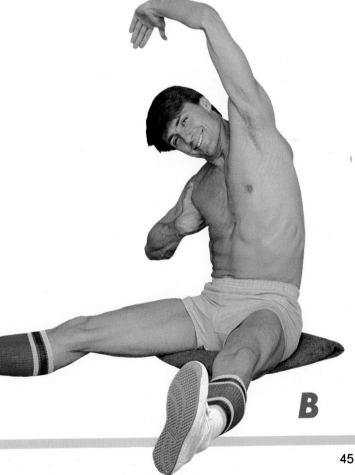

MOUNTAIN CLIMBER

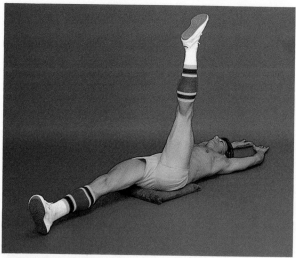

Starting Position

A Sit up, swinging the arms forward and raising the right leg to meet the left leg. Touch fingertips to feet. Return to starting position. Repeat 10 times, alternating leg raised with each sit-up.

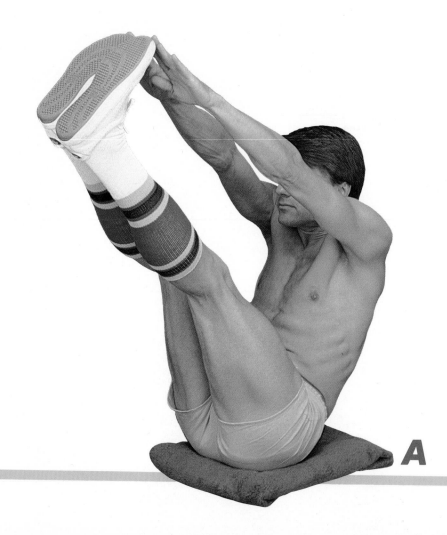

A

JACKKNIFE

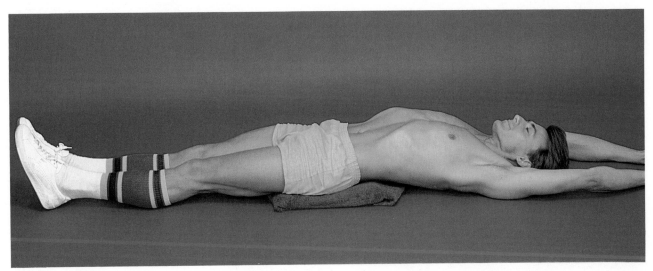

Starting Position

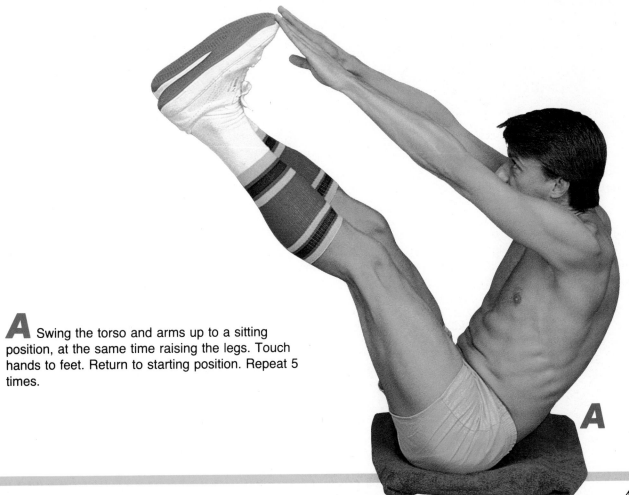

A Swing the torso and arms up to a sitting position, at the same time raising the legs. Touch hands to feet. Return to starting position. Repeat 5 times.

A

POUND THAT FLOOR

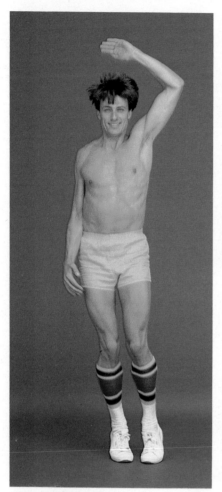
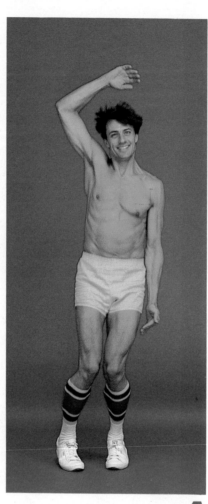

Starting Position

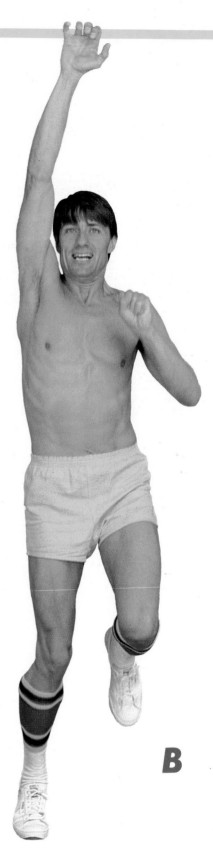

A

A "Ski jump" from side to side for 20 counts: Keeping thighs together, jump to the right and raise right arm. Then jump to the left, raising left arm.

B Run in place for 150 counts, raising opposite arm high with each step.

B

PAY DIRT FOR THE LATERALS

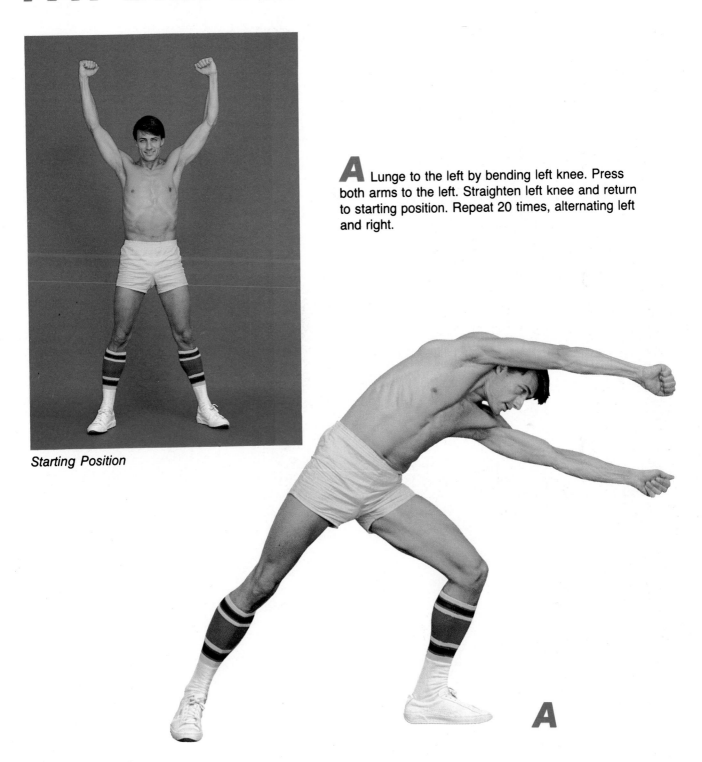

Starting Position

A Lunge to the left by bending left knee. Press both arms to the left. Straighten left knee and return to starting position. Repeat 20 times, alternating left and right.

THE CHALLENGER

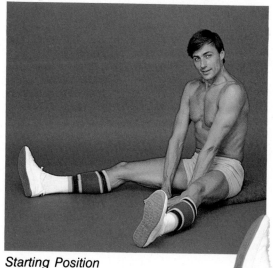

Starting Position

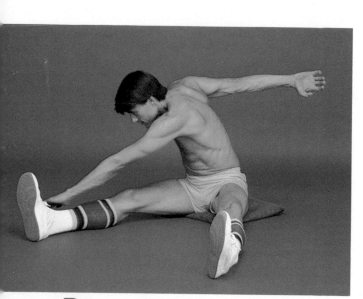

A Raise both legs a few inches off the floor. Hold 3 counts. Raise legs higher and hold 3 counts. Raise legs as high as possible and hold 3 counts. Lower legs to middle level. Hold 3 counts. Lower legs a bit more and hold 3 counts. Lower legs to floor.

B Sit with legs wide apart, arms extended to the sides at shoulder height. Twist and touch right hand to left foot. Return to center and twist to the right. Repeat 10 times. Work those laterals!

50

THE KICK OFF

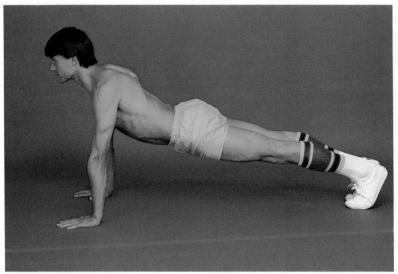

Starting Position

A Swing left leg forward and back. Do not touch the left foot to the floor on the return. Repeat 10 times with each leg.

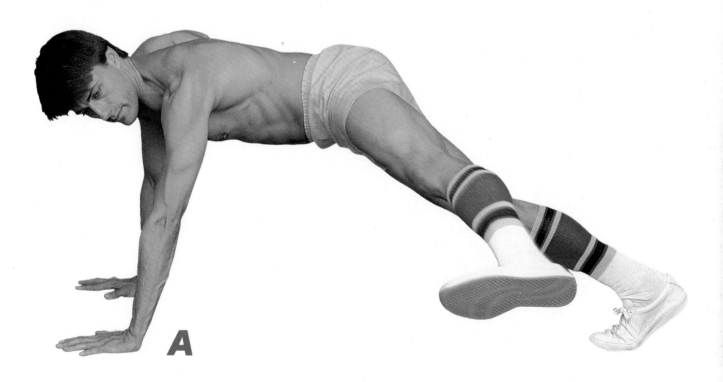

A

PUNT

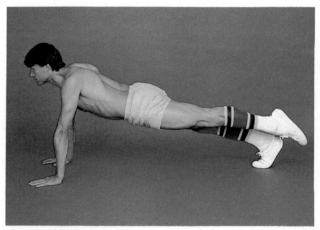

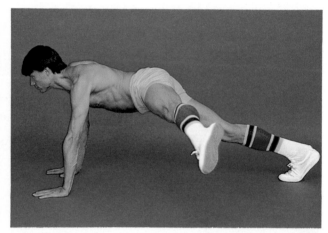

Starting Position

B

A Bend left knee in toward the chest.

B Kick left leg out to the side, then bend knee and bring leg back toward chest. Extend left leg back to starting position, keeping the foot off the floor at all times. Repeat 10 times with each leg.

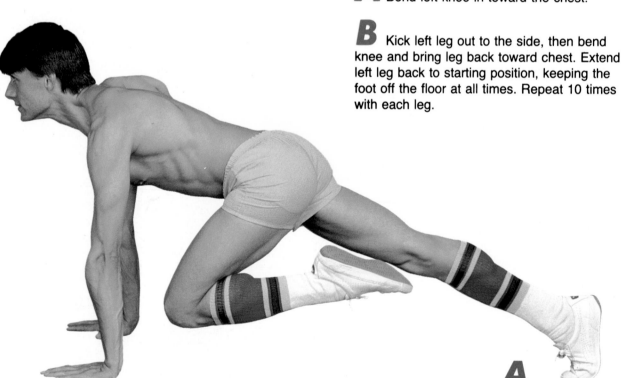

A

STRONGEST

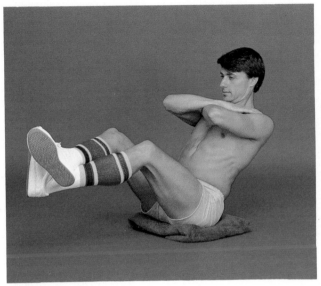
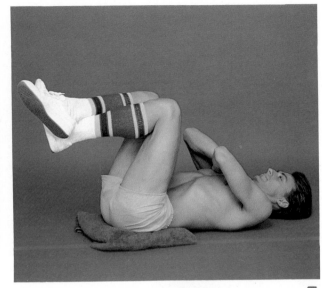

Starting Position

A

A Maintaining leg and arm position, lower the upper torso to the floor and return 10 times.

B Sit with knees apart and soles together. Place hands on the floor by your thighs and allow your head to drop forward. Slowly straighten your back, lift your shoulders, and drop your head back. Take a deep breath and slowly let it out. Repeat 3 times.

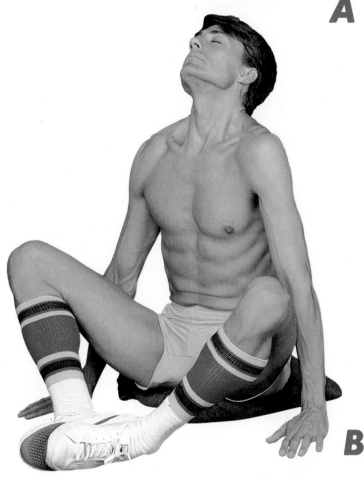

B

TWO-POINT CONVERSION

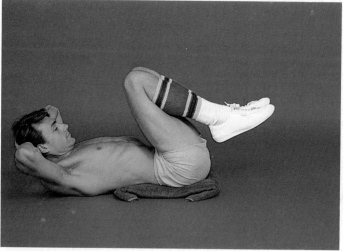

Starting Position

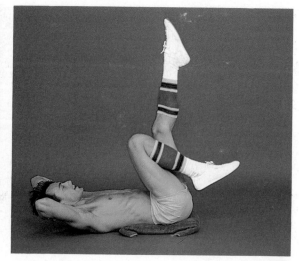

A

A Bicycle-kick straight up for a count of 5.

B Bicycle-kick straight forward for a count of 5, raising your torso up to a sitting position as you do so. Lower your torso to the floor and bicycle-kick up for a count of 5. Do 3 "sit-ups" as you bicycle for a total count of 30 kicks.

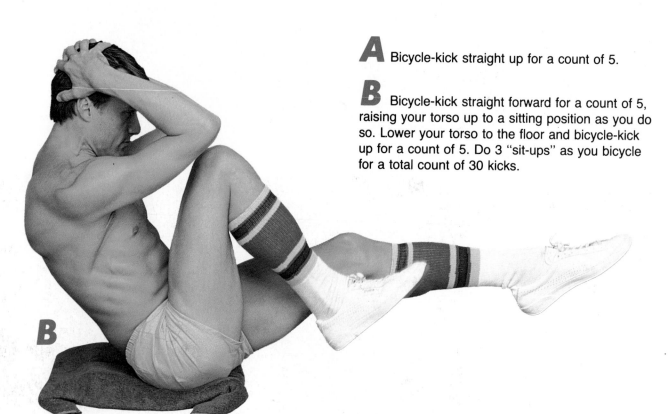

B

POINT AFTER

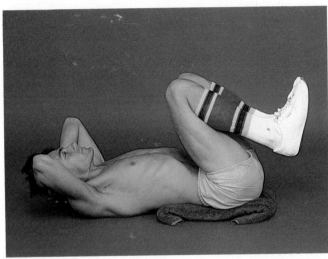

Starting Position

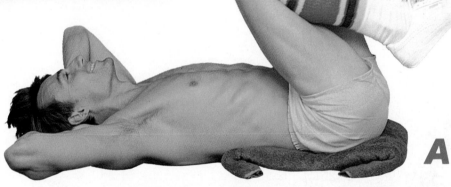

A

A Bicycle-kick straight up for a count of 5.

B Bicycle-kick straight forward for a count of 5. Repeat 3 times.

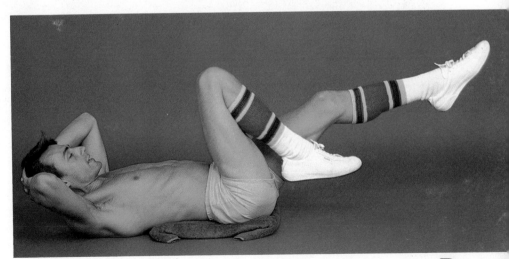

B

THE SWEAT OUT

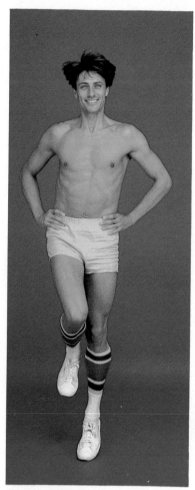
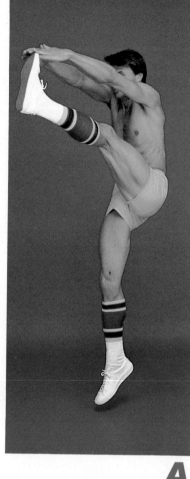

Starting Position

A

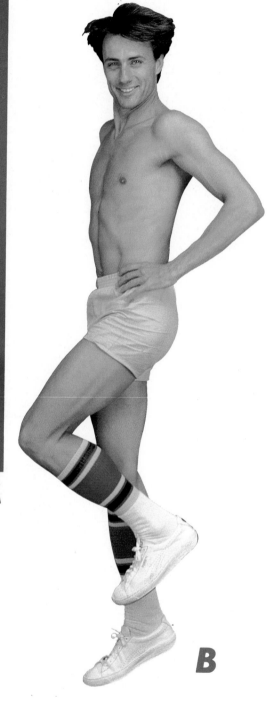

B

A Hop on the right foot and kick the left leg straight forward and up, reaching for left toe with your hands. Repeat the kick 10 times on each leg.

B Hop on the right foot for 25 counts, circling to the right as you hop. Repeat on the left foot. Then run in place for 100 counts.

TOUGH OUT

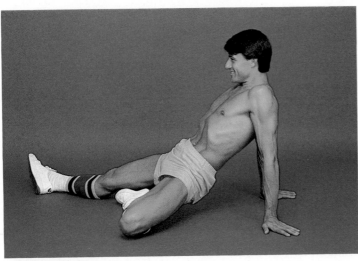

Starting Position

A Raise the right leg from the floor and bring it to a position directly in front of the torso. Do not lower hips to the floor. Lower leg back to starting position. Repeat 10 times on each side.

A

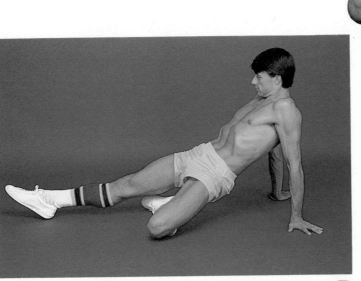

B

B Return to starting position. Raise the right leg as before, but this time lower the leg to the floor directly in front of the body, then raise it back to the center front position before returning it to the starting position. Repeat 10 times on each side.

SIDE SWIPE

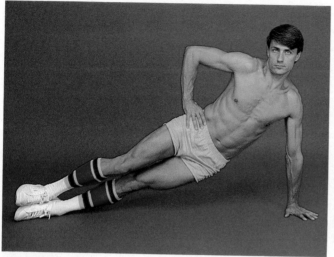

Starting Position

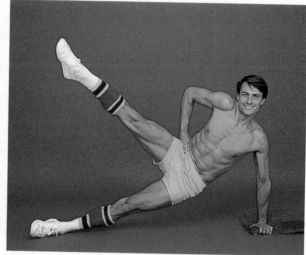

A

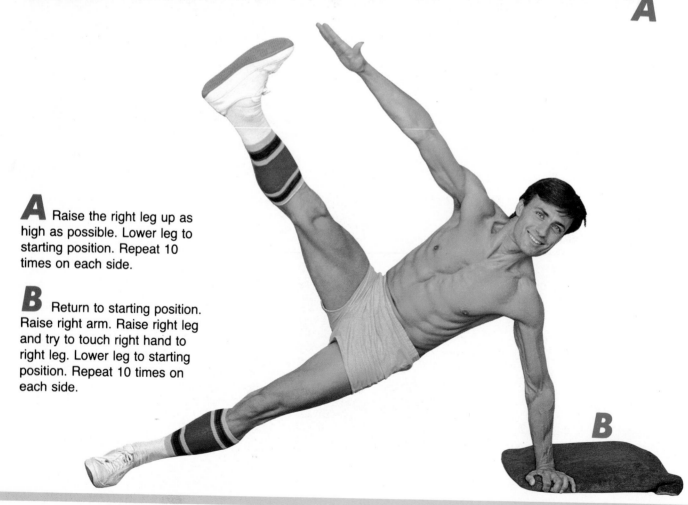

A Raise the right leg up as high as possible. Lower leg to starting position. Repeat 10 times on each side.

B Return to starting position. Raise right arm. Raise right leg and try to touch right hand to right leg. Lower leg to starting position. Repeat 10 times on each side.

B

MIDDLE MULCHER

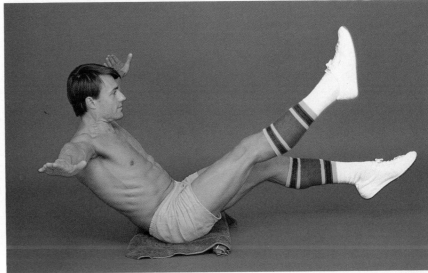

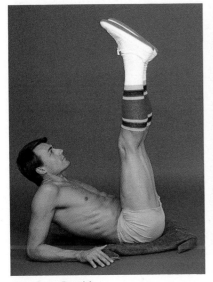

Starting Position

A

A Begin scissors-kicking legs up and down. On the fifth kick, lift arms off floor and extend them out to sides. Kick legs in this position 5 times, then lower arms back to starting position. Repeat 3 times, for a total of 30 scissors kicks.

B Sit on floor, legs extended forward, knees slightly bent. Reach hands forward and try to grasp toes. Hold 5 counts. Release. Repeat 5 times.

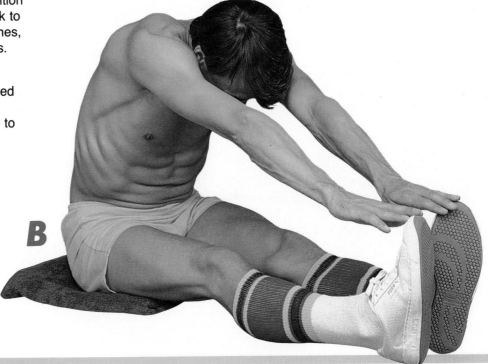

B

EXTRA YARDAGE

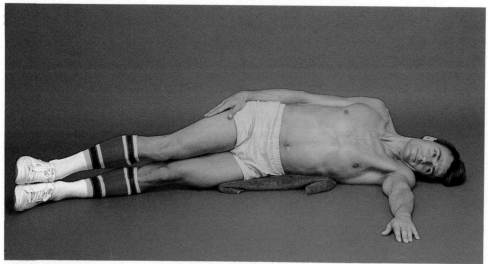

Starting Position

A Swing the right leg forward, trying to touch right foot to left hand. Return to starting position. Repeat 10 times on each side.

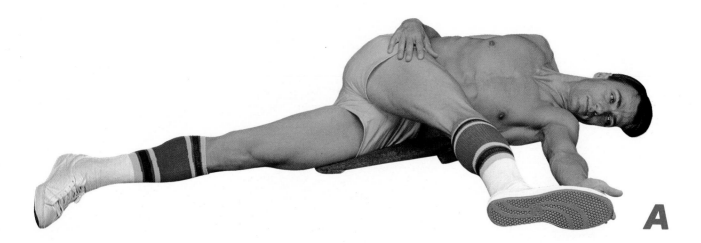

THE LONGEST YARD

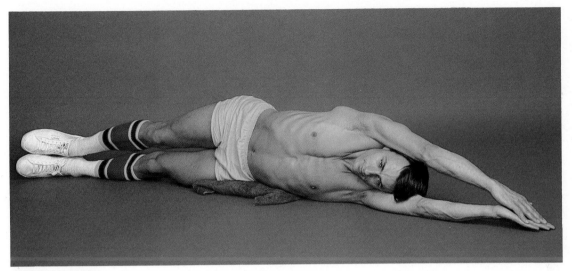

Starting Position

A Raise the right leg and right arm, and touch right toe with right hand. Return to starting position. Repeat 10 times on each side.

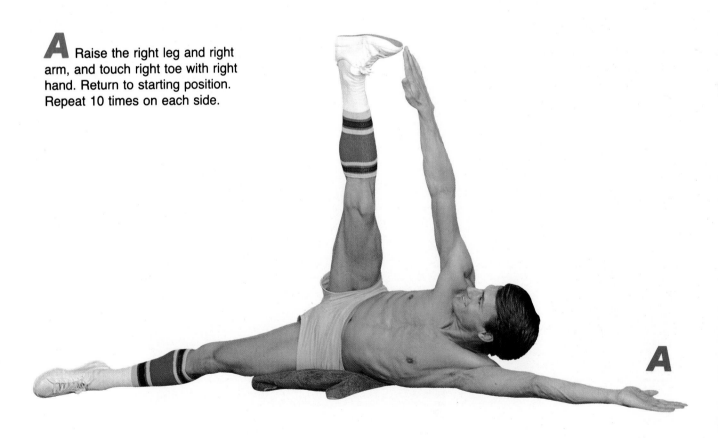

A

TIME OUT

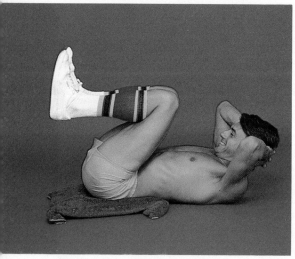

Starting Position

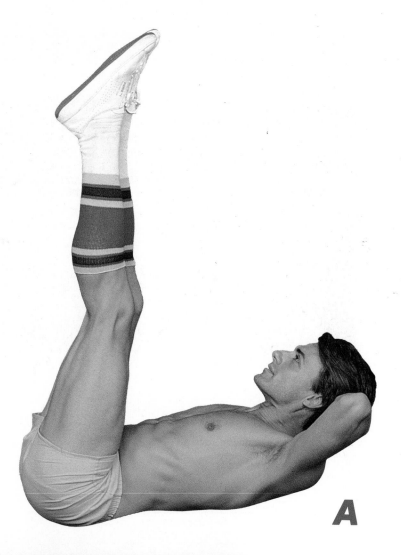

A Extend both legs straight up. Then bend knees in to chest as in starting position.

B Extend legs straight forward, keeping feet off floor. Bend knees in to return to starting position. Repeat 10 times.

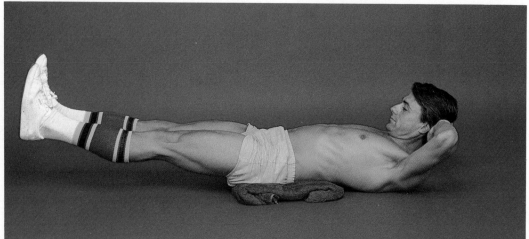

TO THE SHOWERS

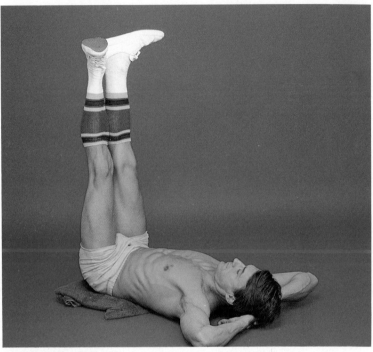

Starting Position

A Keeping heels together and feet turned out, very slowly lower legs to the floor. Try to flatten the back to the floor. Lift legs back to starting position. Repeat 10 times.

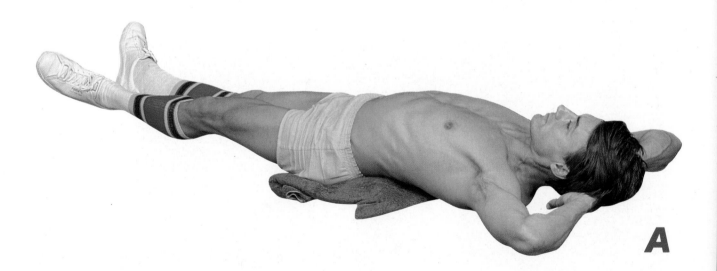

A